How Not To Kill Someone In The ICU

HESHAM A. HASSABALLA, MD, FCCP, FAASM

Faithful Word Press

ISBN: 978-0-9853265-1-7

DEDICATION

To my beloved and beautiful wife, Reem, whose unwavering support has made me who I am. I could not have trod the road I did without her with me every step of the way. Thank you.

CONTENTS

ACKNOWLEDGMENTS

First and foremost, I must thank the Lord my God. Without Him and His unending Love and Mercy, I would be absolutely nothing. I am grateful to all my teachers throughout my medical training, who gave me the medical knowledge I needed to be as successful as I am. I am grateful to all the medical students, nursing students, medical residents and fellows, whose confidence in me as a teacher inspired the writing of this book. Last but not least, I am eternally grateful to Gil Bashe and Dr. Robert Turner, whose counsel, friendship, and mentorship have been invaluable.

PROLOGUE
MY JOURNEY TO THE ICU

Ever since I was a little boy, I have only ever wanted to become a doctor. I "played doctor" growing up and had multiple toy medical sets. I shadowed my uncle, who is an Emergency Medicine physician, more times than I can count, trying to learn the medical lingo and other "tricks of the trade." I even volunteered as a test patient for Family Medicine Residents at Rush Medical College in Chicago, IL, where I wore make up and had to act like a victim of a motor vehicle crash. It was an experience I have never forgotten.

In high school, my community service project was in a hospital, helping get patients water and cleaning IV poles. I also had a summer job cleaning and sterilizing colonoscopes in between patients. When the surgeon would let me hold the biopsy forceps and open and close them to take biopsies, I was on cloud nine. Medicine was truly my dream career, and there was nothing else I saw myself becoming as an adult.

So, after graduating high school, I attended Marquette University for my undergraduate studies. My initial major was biochemistry, because – again – I only wanted to be a doctor, and I figured this is a "good major" for premedical students. One of my co-residents in my dorm, however, convinced me to switch to biomedical engineering. It was a particularly difficult major, and it made my path to medical school that much harder.

But, in 1992, there were practically no jobs in biomedical engineering – it was truly a brand new field – and thus the major was specifically designed for students like me: premed students who wanted an engineering background. Why engineering? Because I was under no illusion that getting into medical school was guaranteed for me, and I wanted to have a good "back up" career in case I could not matriculate into medical school.

Thankfully, I did well enough in my studies to get a good GPA. I took the MCAT in the summer of 1994 and applied later that fall. I only got one interview: Rush Medical College. I was interviewed in February 1995, and I thought it went OK. One month later, in March 1995, I was placed on the wait list.

There is no way I'm getting in, I told myself. And so, throughout the rest of my school year, I totally forgot about medical school. My uncle, the Emergency Medicine physician, kept harassing me to call the school and find out.

"Why?" I asked him. "I'm not getting in."

"Just call them!" he would retort back to me.

So, one morning, I did just that: I called the school.

"Hello! This is Hesham Hassaballa, and I am calling to get my status on the waiting list." I told the woman on the phone.

"Please hold," she told me. Another person came on the phone, and I told them the same thing: "I am calling to get my status on the waiting list." She asked me for my social security number, and I gave it to her. She then sounded confused:

"Hmm…we sent your acceptance letter last Tuesday."

I was dumbfounded. I honestly did not believe her words. Finally mustering the courage to say something, I said: "Huh. I didn't get the letter. Where did you send it?" She gave an old address, *from which I had moved a week or so before.*

"Oh no, I just moved from there. Can you send it to my new address?"

"Sure!" she said. I then asked, because I still did not believe what I just heard, "So, I've been accepted?"

"Uh huh!"

I hung up the phone and screamed out loud. The day about which I had dreamt for literally decades, the day for which had prayed, literally thousands of times, had finally come. I was going to medical school.

I graduated medical school in 1999. Other than finally becoming a doctor and fulfilling my dream, the other best thing about graduating medical school is that I finally no longer felt like a fraud when I called myself "Dr. Hassaballa." You see, in medical school, if I said I was a student, more often than not, they would hang up the phone in my face. So, to get things done, I would call myself "Dr. Hassaballa."

My first month as a doctor, during my internship, was in the Coronary Care Unit, where critically ill heart patients are treated. I still remember the awe I felt when seeing my name, "Hassaballa" next to five patient names on the board in the CCU. Now, it is no longer "pretend"; now, I have real, live people entrusted to my care. The reality was daunting.

But, I loved every minute of it. I knew, for certain, that being a Pulmonary and Critical Care specialist is what I wanted to do for the rest of my life. I told my Chief Residents of my desire, and so they tailored my rotations to give me more months in the ICU than a typical Resident in Internal Medicine. Once in the ICU, I knew I was home.

I just love the ICU: the sickest of the sick, at their most vulnerable, come to the ICU, and it was so cool to aggressively push to try and save them from death. The ICU is fast-paced and unpredictable. You get to perform procedures; you get to behold the evolution of critical illness literally in a matter of hours; and when you help people survive life-threatening illness, the feeling that brings you is truly indescribable.

What's more, in the ICU, I truly feel like a "doctor." As a lung specialist, my only concern is the lungs. Same is true with other specialists, such as Cardiologists, Gastroenterologists, or Cardiac Surgeons. But, in the ICU, I am part Surgeon when I do procedures; I am also part Pulmonologist, Cardiologist, Gastroenterologist,

Endocrinologist, Neurologist, and Internist. I have to understand and manage multiple different organ systems and make sure I can harmonize them as much as possible. It is so awesome.

In addition, when I know that I am going to lose the battle with the critical illness, it is now my chance to help mitigate and reduce the suffering of my patient, to allow my patient to die with dignity. And, I can also help the family who is dealing with the death of their loved one. Truly, in the ICU, I can do good whether my patient lives or dies. That is why I made the ICU the place where I will spend my entire career.

INTRODUCTION
A DAY IN THE LIFE OF AN INTENSIVIST

Even though I love being in the ICU, my career path did not start exclusively in the ICU. My training program was a combined one in which I became a specialist in Pulmonary Medicine, Critical Care Medicine, and Sleep Medicine. It was one of those rare training programs in which I can be eligible to sit for three board examinations. At that time, many – if not most – training programs for Critical Care Medicine were combined with Pulmonary Medicine or another subspecialty. It was not until later that stand-alone Critical Care Medicine programs started to grow in number.

So, after I finished my training, I joined a traditional Pulmonary and Critical Care Medicine private practice. We were "jacks of all trades," simultaneously practicing outpatient Pulmonary Medicine, inpatient Pulmonary Medicine, and inpatient Critical Care Medicine. It was horribly inefficient.

For example, it was not infrequent that I would have to leave a very sick patient in the ICU after seeing them for a few minutes because I had an office full of patients waiting for me. And, after I finished seeing all of those patients in the office, I would travel back and forth between multiple hospitals seeing patients in the ICU and on the medical floor. It was exhausting.

Then, the opportunity to lead an Intensivist program from the ground up presented itself, and it was simply too good to pass up. I made the difficult decision to leave my private practice and run the ICU in which I currently practice. I have not looked back since.

Today, many ICUs have dedicated Critical Care Medicine specialists – whom we call "Intensivists" – who only work and practice in the ICU. It is largely a shift-based practice, where clinicians spend their shift (typically between 7AM and 7PM) and see most if not all of the patients admitted to the ICU. Basically, the Intensivist is the "captain of the ship," but he or she does not practice alone. There is an entire team of clinicians who cares for the patient, including (most importantly) the ICU nurse, respiratory therapist, physical therapist, occupational therapist, care manager, nutritionist, pharmacist, and many others.

A typical day can start by getting a "sign out" or a report from the clinician who was covering the ICU during the night shift about any new patients who were admitted or any major overnight events that occurred with one or more of the ICU patients. Then, the Intensivist will go from room to room and see all of the patients admitted to the ICU. Once this is done, in many ICUs the Intensivist will run multidisciplinary care rounds, where the entire treatment team comes together and discusses the plan of care of each patient in the ICU.

Once rounds are finished, the Intensivist may need to perform various procedures that the patients need The Intensivist may need to discuss the care of the patients with other specialists, such as Cardiologists or Nephrologists. The Intensivist may have one or more family conferences to discuss overall goals of care of one or more ICU patients. The Intensivist will have to find time to document in the medical record on all the patients he or she has seen throughout the day, all the while seeing any new admissions that may come to the ICU during the shift.

Some ICUs are what we call "closed," where the Intensivist has full control over who gets admitted to the ICU, which specialist gets consulted for the ICU patients, and when a patient is discharged from the ICU. Other ICUs are "open" models, where any clinician can admit to the ICU, and the Intensivist is consulted to coordinate the care of the patient. The model chosen depends on the individual factors and culture of each hospital. In my ICU, it is an "open" model with a mandatory consultation of the Intensivist, and it works very well.

I have been practicing in the ICU for more than twenty years. I have seen and experienced a lot, especially during the COVID-19 pandemic. Yes, the job of an Intensivist may seem daunting. On many days it is, but it is an awesome job, and throughout my years I have learned so many lessons, and I now want to share those lessons with you.

Reflecting over my time in the ICU, I have discerned several principles of practice, what I like to call my "Top Rules of the ICU." I always teach these rules to any student or resident who rotates with me in my ICU. I have found these "Top Rules" to have helped me tremendously in my practice, and it is my sincere hope and prayer that it will help you as well. And these "Top Rules" apply whether you are a nurse, doctor, resident, or student who is going to do one rotation and never again see the ICU or – like I did – decide to make the ICU the place of your career.

CHAPTER 1
ICU RULE NUMBER ONE

"*Dr. Hassaballa!!!! I need you in here right now!!!*"

I have lost count of the number of times I have heard those words coming from an ICU room. It is the voice of the ICU nurse, who needs my assistance with a patient who has suddenly deteriorated.

One night in the ICU, a patient who had just had open heart surgery was getting a little agitated and confused. With all of the tubes and lines in his body, if he were to pull one of them out, it could lead to serious disaster. What's more, he has a large incision down the front of his chest, and if he uses his arms, that could also cause serious damage. So, I prescribed a medication in his IV to calm him down.

Suddenly, almost as soon as he got it, he turned blue. He was clearly not breathing. There was no one else in the room but me, and so it was my turn to scream out of the room: "Call a Code!!!"

"Calling a Code" means having the hospital operator announce overhead, "Code Blue," which usually indicates that a patient has suffered cardiac arrest. "Code Blue" called overhead means, "I need help from anyone and everyone who can come."

A sudden airway emergency is one of, if not my number one, nightmare in the ICU. This patient was clearly not breathing, and I had to quickly intubate him, which means to insert a breathing tube into his airway to prevent him from getting permanent brain damage from lack of oxygen. My legs were shaking, I was so nervous.

Thankfully, I was able to place a tube into his throat quickly. His heart never stopped. It turns out that the medication I gave can rarely – extremely rarely – cause spasm of the vocal cords. The patient did well after this, and he came off the ventilator the following day.

I had another patient who – attempting suicide – drank a commercially available weed killer. This causes severe injury of the mucosa of the mouth and throat, and his whole mouth was bloody. Unfortunately, his oxygen levels started to decrease despite giving him high amounts of supplemental oxygen through his nose and mouth. Unfortunately, it was time to intubate.

All I could see was blood. There was so much bleeding from the mucosal injury that I literally could not see the vocal cords. And, to make matters worse, I had given him sedation so I could place the tube into his throat without him fighting me. My legs were shaking, I was so nervous.

Then, as I was trying to find the airway, his oxygen levels started to decrease and decrease fast. Nurses all around me were screaming, "Oxygen is in the 70s!!!" So, I decided to stop and give him more oxygen by bag-mask valve. It was not working, and now, his heart rate started to decrease as well. So, I grabbed the airway tube and tried again, with both his oxygen levels and heart rate low. Again, all I could see was blood, and he was about to suffer cardiac arrest. I saw some bubbles, and I went toward the bubbles. Thankfully, the airway was there, and I placed the tube into the trachea. Both his oxygen levels and heart rate quickly recovered. My legs were still shaking for several minutes after the crisis abated.

During my Fellowship training, I was on the Pulmonary Medicine service, and we were consulted to perform a bronchoscopy (camera test in the lung) to diagnose possible sarcoidosis in a very sick man in the Coronary Care Unit. The bronchoscopy started out smoothly, and we proceeded to take biopsies of the lung tissue. The first biopsy had a little bit of bleeding, and I looked to my Attending Physician and asked whether we should proceed. He nodded in the affirmative.

I took the second biopsy, and there was even more bleeding this time around. Once again, I looked to my Attending Physician and asked if we should proceed with the next biopsy. Once again, he nodded in the affirmative. So, I took the third biopsy. This time, the bleeding was *even worse*. All I could see was blood on my screen, and I could not stop it.

So, I pulled the camera out of his lungs and sat him up. He was coughing up blood and sedated (from the medicine I just gave him for the procedure). His oxygen levels then began to decrease, all the while continuing to cough up blood. Thus, we decided to intubate him, so he could properly oxygenate. We called overhead to let people know that we were , ntubating him, and my colleagues from the ICU came down to be present and help if necessary.

The intubation went well, but his oxygen levels did not improve. Then, suddenly, my colleague in the ICU asked, "Is there a pulse?" I felt for one…and I could not feel one.

"CODE BLUE…BRONCHOSCOPY" was called overhead.

We started CPR. I was absolutely horrified. Even though he was sick, he was nevertheless awake and alert and very much alive before the bronchoscopy. Now, he was pulseless, and we were coding him. After working on him, his pulse did come back, but he was in terrible shock. He was on a ventilator, sedated, and on multiple medications to support his blood pressure. I seriously thought he was going to die that day.

"Who did the bronchoscopy?" asked a frustrated senior resident in the CCU.

"I did," I said, and I could feel the tremendous irritation betrayed by her face, because now, she had to deal with a horribly sick patient who suffered a complication of an elective procedure that I did. Oh, and it was Friday the 13th, by the way.

The rest of the day, I could not think straight. I had no appetite. I thought I killed that patient. The following morning, I went straight to the CCU to check up on him, half-expecting his room to be empty. To my great surprise and elation, he was not only alive, but he had pulled out the breathing tube on his own, nexpectedly. I asked him, "How do you feel?"

"Like shit," he replied.

Those two words made me happier than I could ever have been, because he understood what I said and replied, indicating that he survived the complication without significant brain damage. I was so relieved he was okay.

All of these stories highlight the absolute importance of **ICU Rule Number One**:

DON'T PANIC

In the ICU, at any moment, a patient can suddenly deteriorate and deteriorate quickly. During the initial wave of the COVID pandemic in 2020, the patients we saw in the hospital and ICU were super sick, and they deteriorated super quickly. At any moment, a patient outside of the ICU can suddenly suffer a cardiac arrest or respiratory complication, and we are called to respond and help tend to the patient. The absolute first thing I must do is **NOT panic**.

When I was an intern, my senior resident told me, when a critical situation arises, to "check your own pulse first." When we panic, we freeze in fear, and we are liable to not think clearly and logically. In fact, once I asked a resident who was rotating with me in the ICU to run a Code Blue to which we both responded. He simply froze. So, I (gently) pushed him aside and took over running the Code.

During crisis situations, it is not uncommon for everyone else in the room to panic. It is frequently a chaotic scene, with multiple people speaking at the same time and talking over each other. People are visibly rattled and uncomfortable. It is *absolutely essential* that the leader – you – is calm, cool, and collected. That way, you can think clearly about what happened, why it happened, and what you need to do about it.

Yes, the patient may die. Yes, the situation may get worse, despite your initial intervention. Yes, the patient's condition may progress to cardiac arrest – like that patient upon which I performed the bronchoscopy – but it does not matter. It is *absolutely essential*, nay life-saving, that you do not panic.

Which brings me to my next ICU RULES:

ICU Rule Number Two: DON'T PANIC
ICU Rule Number Three: DON'T PANIC
ICU Rule Number Four: DON'T PANIC
ICU Rule Number Five: DON'T PANIC

During COVID, we had to intubate a patient because his oxygen levels were not sustainable, and the patient needed a ventilator. I called my Anesthesiologist colleague to do the intubation, because it was a tenuous situation, and I needed an airway expert to do the procedure (another one of my ICU Rules). After he placed the tube into the patient's throat, the patient's oxygen level decreased to 8%.

Now, this level is normally not compatible with life. Most patients' hearts will stop well before the oxygen levels decrease that low. But, with COVID, for some reason which I still do not understand, they can tolerate oxygen levels that low. The Anesthesiologist was panicking. I put my hand on his shoulder and said, "It's all good bruh…it will come up eventually." It did, and that patient actually went on to survive COVID and leave the ICU alive (one of very few that month). The key for me was to not panic.

Now, could I be panicking on the inside? ABSOLUTELY. We are dealing with life and death here. My bronchoscopy patient's heart stopped after I did a biopsy in his lungs. The suicide patient was about to suffer a cardiac arrest. The heart surgery patient stopped breathing and was turning blue before my eyes. This is scary stuff. In each of these situations, I was *most definitely* panicking…on the inside.

On the outside, however, I was as calm as can be. In fact, it may even look as if I am callous, uncaring, and disinterested. I assure you I am not. I am actively staying as calm as possible so I can think clearly about what I need to do to try and save my patient's life. I cannot stress this rule enough, which is why it is my top five Rules of the ICU.

Don't panic. It literally can become a matter of life and death.

CHAPTER 2
ICU RULE NUMBER SIX

It was New Year's Eve, and I was tasked with working the night shift. The ER called me about a patient who required admission to the ICU. She was brought to the ER comatose. When I looked up the patient, I recognized her immediately. Several weeks beforehand, she had a ruptured intestine, and her abdomen was full of infection and pus. She needed surgery, and she was in the hospital a long time. So, when she came back to the ER comatose, I was absolutely certain what she had: sepsis.

Sepsis is organ failure as a result of the body's reaction to infection. I thought, given how bad her abdomen looked, she must have had an infection in her abdomen again causing her to become comatose. I didn't need a CT scan to prove it. The Emergency Medicine team, however, was also worried that she may have ingested a toxic alcohol like methanol (wood alcohol) or ethylene glycol (antifreeze). I puffed in indignation.

"She has sepsis!" I nearly screamed. "I know this patient well! Get the antibiotics! Give her fluids! She is septic!"

My colleagues in the ER were like, *Dude, Hassaballa, RELAX!* I was hearing none of it, however. And when they called Poison Control, I rolled my eyes. *What is wrong with these people?* I said to myself. *She is clearly septic.*

In the process of admitting her to the ICU, I spoke with the

Poison Control representative. I was adamant, agitated and nearly screaming to him on the phone, that she was septic. He calmly explained to me that, whenever patients with such severe acid levels in the blood present to the emergency department, it is very important to make sure there is not a toxic alcohol ingestion present. I rolled my eyes. "She is septic!" I said again (probably for the hundredth time). He said, "Well, that is our recommendation." I, once again, puffed under my breath and thought to myself, *Dumb Toxicology Fellow or ER Resident can't tell me what to do!*

As I was writing admission orders to the ICU, I ordered a CT scan of abdomen, partly to prove to everyone that I was right, and they were wrong. And, I also (quietly) ordered a blood level of ethylene glycol, also to prove that I was right and they were wrong. When I looked up the CT of the abdomen, I was dumbfounded. I could not believe my eyes: the CT of the abdomen was *totally normal.* If I had not known her history, I would have never guessed that she had an infection weeks before.

Then the ethylene glycol level came back: it was positive. I had to come back to the hospital to place a catheter in her vein so she could get emergency dialysis. It turned out that the Poison Control representatives were right, the Emergency Room colleagues were right, and I was wrong: she did indeed ingest antifreeze to attempt suicide. She received several treatments of dialysis and greatly improved. After she recovered, she admitted to attempting suicide with antifreeze, and she was discharged to an inpatient behavioral health facility.

She would have died if I didn't start dialysis on her. She would have died if I succumbed to my ego and didn't order the ethylene glycol level. Whenever I have students or residents in my ICU, I always recount this story to remind myself, first and foremost, and them of my **ICU Rule Number Six**:

YOUR EGO CAN BE DANGEROUS

It should not come as a shock that doctors, especially, can have strong egos. We are largely respected in society, respected in the hospitals and healthcare settings in which we work, and we are leaders in our respective domains. We give orders, and most of the time – especially in the ICU – the orders are carried out without question. Moreover, most of the time, those orders help patients get better and survive critical illness.

That power, however, can quickly corrupt. That respect can easily go to someone's head. It is a constant risk of our profession. And that inflated ego can kill people. We need to squash that ego into a pulp and not let it interfere with our patient care in the ICU.

We should not bristle when a nurse, medical student, resident, respiratory therapist, or even fellow asks a question that seems silly to us. We should not dismiss the suggestions of those who have less experience or knowledge than we do. Everyone has a different perspective, a different way to look at the same case, and that perspective can give us insight and help us better care for our patient.

I shudder to think what could have happened if I had succumbed to my ego and not ordered the ethylene glycol level. Like I said, she could have died. I have never forgotten that lesson, and it is why I teach it to everyone who rotates in my ICU and why I included it in my Top Rules for the ICU.

CHAPTER 3
ICU RULE NUMBER SEVEN

"*Call a Code!!!!*"

I have also lost count of the number of times I have spoken these three words in the course of my career in the ICU. When we "call a code," we are asking the hospital operator to announce overhead, so the entire hospital can hear, "Code Blue, Room XXX." This means that the patient has suffered cardiac arrest, and we need all hands on deck to help care for the patient. Even if I am in the ICU, if a patient suffers cardiac arrest, we are "calling a code." Remember that patient that had vocal cord spasm from a medication? I called a code, even though I had full control of the airway and the clinical situation. I needed the help, just in case something went wrong.

As part of the care we deliver in the ICU, many times we need to perform a procedure we call a "central line." This is where we insert, most often using ultrasound guidance, a special long IV into a large vein in the chest, neck, or sometimes groin. This special IV is required if we are giving powerful blood pressure medications called vasopressors, or giving multiple medications at once. It is much more robust IV than the smaller ones we insert into the veins of the hands or arms.

Now, I have placed hundreds and hundreds of these lines over my career. I can practically do them with my eyes closed. At times, however, I can have difficulty placing these central lines. It may be due to the patient's veins, previous surgeries, or any other reason. So, when this occurs, I call my Interventional Radiology colleagues to help me. And almost always, they come to the bedside and place the line with absolutely no difficulty at all.

This same situation has happened to me when placing a special IV in the artery called an arterial line, which allows me to monitor blood pressure much more accurately. I can try and try for a very long time, and then I call my Anesthesia colleagues to help, and they – again – place the line with absolutely no difficulty. This illustrates my **ICU Rule Number Seven**:

YOU ARE NEVER TOO COOL TO ASK FOR HELP

When I try and try and can't get a procedure, and then my colleague comes and performs it so easily that I look like a novice, yeah – my ego gets bruised a little. Who cares. Rather than keep sticking the patient with a needle dozens of times because, "I can do this!", I will acknowledge my attempt and then call those colleagues who also have good experience in performing these procedures for help. The same is true if I know – right from the outset – that someone with more experience needs to perform a procedure.

This happened multiple times during the COVID-19 pandemic. Just like central lines, I have placed hundreds of breathing tubes in patients' lungs. I can also practically do this with my eyes closed. At the same time, when we had to place breathing tubes in COVID-19 patients, there is very little time to waste before oxygen levels become dangerously low. If I think that I may have even the slightest difficulty with an airway, I am calling my Anesthesiology colleagues to place the airway instead of me. I am not going to jeopardize someone's health to make a point that "I can do this!" That is just dumb and reckless.

This same rule, you are never too cool to ask for help, applies to consultants in the ICU. In many ICUs, the Intensivists – or Critical Care Medicine specialists – are in charge of patient management. This is how most training programs in Critical Care Medicine nowadays are also set up. We manage every aspect of the care: the ventilators, the antibiotics, the medications, the procedures, and most everything else. Typically, we do not call other specialists to help manage cases in the ICU.

Yet, sometimes, we do need the help from other specialists.

Sometimes, we do need help from an Infectious Disease specialist when we are dealing with infections. Sometimes, we do need help from a Cardiologist when we are dealing with a heart condition, such as an acute myocardial infarction. Sometimes, we do need help from an Endocrinologist to manage complex diabetic patients. Can we handle it all on our own? Most probably. Yet, Critical Care Medicine is a team sport, and we should never be too cool to ask for help from other consultants in the appropriate circumstance.

Given that Critical Care Medicine is a team sport, it also means that we should never be too cool to ask for help from other clinicians who can offer their expertise in the ICU. For example, I am sure I can do a fine job ordering enteral or IV nutrition. I am sure I can look it up and order the right formulation for the patient, but I have Certified Nutritionists who round in the hospital every day. So, I ask them for their recommendations when it comes to nutrition for my ICU patients.

Yes, I can look up which medications to order for my patients, but I also have a dedicated Pharmacist in my ICU. So, why not take advantage of their expertise? They monitor all the medications my patients are prescribed, make sure I do not make a mistake with respect to dosing, ensure that the medications I order do not interact with other medications, and many other things. I can't do my job well without them.

The same thing goes with the Respiratory Therapists, who are part and parcel of any good functioning ICU. They are not "knob turners" on the ventilator. Anybody can do that. Rather, they are highly skilled clinicians who understand the respiratory system better than most other clinicians, and they use that knowledge to help a patient breathe well on mechanical ventilation. I also can't do my job well without them.

I feel the same way about the Physical Therapists, Occupational Therapists, Chaplains, Case Managers, and others who help care for our patients in the ICU. Each of them plays such an important role, and while – yes – as the Critical Care Specialist, I am leading the care, I cannot do my job properly without countless others in the ICU who have expertise, knowledge, and knowhow to help a patient navigate critical illness in the easiest and safest manner possible.

No, I can't do it all myself. Sometimes, despite trying my hardest, I just can't get a procedure done, and someone else comes and does it flawlessly. Who cares. We are dealing with life and death here in the ICU. Given that fact, we should never be too cool to call for help when our patients need it.

CHAPTER 4
ICU RULE NUBMER EIGHT

"Doctor? I am sorry to bother you, but the patient's potassium level is 3.4. Do you want to do anything about it?"

Almost always, I get this phone call in the middle of the night from an ICU nurse caring for a patient in the ICU. And, almost always, it is about a slightly abnormally low potassium level. First of all, ICU Nurses, please stop saying, "*Sorry to bother you.*" If you were *truly sorry* to bother me, you would not have called me in the first place, but I digress…

There are myriad abnormal numbers in the ICU: heart rate numbers, laboratory study numbers, blood pressure numbers, to name a few. Some of the numbers are significant, and others are insignificant. The challenge is to determine which numbers matter, and which numbers do not matter. There is an urge on the part of some clinicians to act on every single abnormal number, and if I do not, it seems that I do not care about treating the patient.

For example, we were transferring a COVID patient to a University medical center for possible ECMO (external heart-lung machine). His heart rate was abnormally high. The nurse called me about it, and I did not want to do anything about it. It was likely a reaction to us moving him to the transport equipment, and it would likely get better without any intervention. The nurse called me again about the same number, and again, I declined to do anything about the number. After the nurse called me a third time, I ordered a mediation to slow the heart rate down. And, as a result, the blood pressure went down (which I knew could happen and was part of the reason why I declined to do anything about the heart rate in the first place). Therefore, I had to give another medicine to increase the blood pressure, counteracting the medication I gave to slow down the heart rate. It was a frustrating exercise in futility.

Another time, I got a frantic call from an ICU nurse before my shift started. I called back, worried that it was a serious patient emergency that demanded my immediate attention. The breathless nurse told me that the patient's – you guessed it – potassium level was 3.4 (which is barely abnormal), and no one was calling her back. Flabbergasted, I responded that this is not an emergency, and I have never lost a patient from a potassium level of 3.4. She said, "It's all good now as I got a hold of the Nephrologist."

This brings me to my **ICU Rule Number Eight**:

TREAT THE PATIENT

Treat the patient, not the number. Sometimes, a number may be abnormal, but it does not matter to the overall patient's well-being. Or, treating the number may actually do more harm than good, such as my COVID patient being transferred to the University. We need to look at the overall patient and decide whether or not a specific abnormal number is clinically significant.

For example, many patients in the ICU have abnormally elevated heart rates, and we are frequently notified about these abnormally elevated heart rates. Yet, what does the high heart rate mean? Do they have a fever? Are they complaining of pain? Is it just part of their disease process? Patients with diabetic ketoacidosis frequently have elevated heart rates and respiratory rates. Yet, if we treat the underlying DKA, the elevated heart rate and respiratory rate will resolve on its own, without any specific intervention or medication. If I treat the elevated respiratory rate, for example, by intubating them and placing them on a ventilator, that could kill the patient. Not every abnormal number needs an intervention.

When I was in private practice as a Pulmonologist, I would frequently encounter patients with an abnormal CT scan of the chest, showing a nodule. The nodule could be cancer. First question I ask, however, is this:

"If this nodule is cancer, will you want surgery?"

My patient answers, "No."

"If this nodule is cancer, will you want chemotherapy?"

"No," says my patient again.

"If this nodule is cancer, will you want radiation?"

"No," says my patient a third time.

"So, don't worry about the nodule. Have a great day."

This is treating the patient, and not the "number," which in this instance was an abnormal imaging study. If the patient does not want to treat the abnormal finding, even if it is cancer, and they understand the implications of not treating the abnormal finding, then that is their right; that is their goal of care, and it is our responsibility as clinicians to stay within the goals of care of our patients.

As another example, I have a deviated nasal septum. It is an "S" shape. I cannot breathe at night without a nasal strip. I have been offered surgery to fix the deviated septum, and the surgery is very low risk, but I ask the surgeon, what is the chance that I could permanently lose my smell and taste? "Less than 1%," he says. No thanks. That is too high of a risk for me.

I LOVE to eat. It is one of the joys of life for me. If I can't smell or taste food, I'd rather be dead. And so, I would rather continue to not breathe through my nose than risk losing – however unlikely – my smell and taste as a result of a septoplasty surgery. That is my goal of care.

Goals of care are extremely important when it comes to treating patients in the ICU. It is one of the other aspects of the ICU Rule of "Treat the Patient." Whenever a patient is admitted to the ICU, we ask the patient about "code status." This is asking the patient, or their loved one, what we should do if the patient "codes," or suffers respiratory or cardiac arrest. A "Full Code," means that – if the heart or breathing stops – we will perform CPR, shock the heart if necessary, and place a breathing tube into the airway and place the patient on a ventilator. The opposite of "Full Code" is "DNR," which means "Do Not Resuscitate." This directs the treatment team to NOT perform CPR, or shock the heart, or place the patient on a ventilator. Asking about "code status" is a variation of the question, "Do you want me to 'do everything'?". Even though we ask this question all the time, it is exactly the wrong question to ask.

Asking a patient, or their loved ones if the patient cannot answer for himself or herself, if we should "do everything" connotes that we are OK with watching a patient die and not doing anything about it. That's not what we do in the ICU. We do not sip our coffee and just "watch people die."

The question to ask is this: what is your goal of care? "Doing everything" may mean you may die on a machine. So, we should ask our patients, "Do you want to die on a machine? Do you want to die with us pounding on your chest, shocking your heart, and on a ventilator breathing for you?" A question I always ask my patients' families, when discussing goals of care, is this: "If your family member stood where I am standing and saw themselves, what would they say?"

The answers to those questions are absolutely essential. It defines what I call the "patients' red lines," ones which I should never cross. If a patient wants to live at all costs; if a patient wants to die on a machine, then I will fulfill their wish, regardless of how I feel about it. That is their goal of care, and working for the patient, I need to fulfill their goals of care.

I suspect, and my experience treating patients in the ICU has shown me, that most people do not want to die on a machine. Most patients do not want to die with someone pounding on their chest or shocking their heart. CPR is not nice and clean like it is on TV shows and movies. It is brutal. It is forceful by design. We break ribs. We break breastbones. It is very painful. Most people do not want to die that way. So, we need to make sure they understand what the implications of "doing everything" truly are.

Just because I can do something, does not mean I should do it. Sometimes, the burdens of aggressive intervention come to outweigh their benefits. Sometimes, aggressive intervention only prolongs the suffering of the patient. Sometimes, there are things that are *worse* than death. We see this *all the time* in the ICU, and we saw this *all the time* with COVID patients. At that point, we need to pause and clarify goals of care. Do they want to live their last days on a machine? Do they want to be fed through a tube? If the answer is no, then we need to stop, even if that means the patient will die.

Of course, for a temporary illness, it is absolutely appropriate to be as aggressive as possible. It is why we are the ICU in the first place: to aggressively intervene to try and prevent critical illness from killing a patient. And that aggressive intervention can be painful and difficult, with tubes and lines inserted in every orifice in the body. During COVID, we did this on countless patients. And it is appropriate to be aggressive even if the patient is technically "DNR."

"DNR" is not "DNT," or "Do Not Treat." "DNR" just means that, if the heart stops, we should allow natural death. In fact, some hospitals have changed "DNR" to "AND," or "Allow Natural Death." I like to say this: "If the heart stops, that tells me that God wants them more than I do. So, who am I to stand in the way by pounding on his chest and shocking the heart?"

This brings me to another point, and it is related to treating the patient. I am a man of deep faith. I am not even close to the standards to which I aspire every day, and at the same time, I will die trying to be the best believer I can be. It is impossible that I leave my faith at the door of the ICU; it is part and parcel of who I am, the air which I breathe. Every day, as I walk into the hospital before my shift, I say this prayer: "in Your Name, The Healer, do I begin, Lord my God, and in Your Name, The Healer, do I finish, Lord my God."

Not infrequently do patients' families say to me: "We are believers." Not infrequently do my patients themselves say to me, "I believe in God." It does not scare me, or make me uncomfortable in the least. On the contrary, my response is: "I am a believer, too. I also believe in God."

In fact, our shared belief in the Precious Beloved is an asset, not a liability. We come from the same Fountainhead of Life; we share in the Warmth of His Grace; we bask in the Light of His Love. And so, when my patient or their family says they are believers, I welcome it wholeheartedly. And I am comfortable with the language of faith. I understand its frame of reference, and of all the situations of life, critical illness is one in which the flame of faith – even if long extinguished – frequently is rekindled anew.

We doctors should not shy away from faith. If it would be of benefit, we should share our faith and spirituality. Some of my colleagues have prayed with their patients; others have offered counsel within the same faithful frame of reference. That is why I am comfortable saying, "If his or her heart stops, despite everything we are doing, then that is God telling me that He wants him or her back more than I do. Why, then, should I stand in the way?"

I recently saw a nurse ask for a moment of silence after a patient did not survive cardiac arrest. I was so moved by this that I have started doing it myself whenever I run a "Code Blue," and the patient does not survive. I wrote a prayer – in the form of a poem – to honor organ donors, and I try to read it whenever we honor a patient on their way to donate organs to others (see appendix).

My faith strengthens me as a physician. It was solace for me through all those dark days of the pandemic. And, I pray, that my faith makes me a better physician for all those entrusted to my care.

That does not mean that I would ever – ever – impose my religious faith on anyone else, most especially my patients. That would be unethical and inexcusable. My patients' beliefs, values, and preferences may not align with my own, but it is my duty to practice within the red lines of the beliefs, values, and preferences of my patients.

At the same time, my faith and spirituality allow me to connect on another, deeper level with my patients and their loved ones. It helps me be more compassionate. And, if my faith allows me to be a better instrument of God's Healing Presence, then that is something that should be embraced and celebrated. It is another way I am able to "Treat the Patient."

But, again, once the burdens of treatment outweigh the benefits; once the burdens of treatment cross the patient's red lines, then we must stop. None of us knows when we are going to die. None of us knows what will be the ultimate cause of our death. None of that is under our control.

What is under our control, however, are the terms of our death. Everyone deserves a death with dignity, without pain, with loved ones around him or her. We must ensure that, if our patient's death is inevitable, the death is on our patient's – not mine or even the family's – own terms. It is part of my job as an ICU physician.

When patient a comes in trying to die from critical illness, and we work and work to prevent that death and succeed; when we watch a patient walk out of our ICU after nearly dying a few days before, it brings a joy that is truly indescribable. It is why I became a doctor, especially an ICU doctor, in the first place.

That said, if I can also give my patient – one whom I know will die despite everything I have done – a death with dignity; if I can give my patient a death on his or her own terms, that brings me joy as well.

We lost a very young man to COVID-19. We tried so hard to save him, but unfortunately, the disease destroyed his lungs to the point of no return. In 30 days, COVID did as much destruction to that poor man's lungs as would 30 years of smoking. When we realized this, we spoke to his wife about the inevitable death of her husband and how he would want to spend his last days. She indicated that he would not want to die on a machine, and so we withdrew care and made sure he died with comfort, with his wife at his side. A few weeks later, she sent us a note of thanks. She ended it like this:

> *Thank you for allowing him to leave this Earth with dignity and care. You'll never know what an impact you've had on me. Again, thank you for your service.*

I nearly broke down in tears when I read that.

The ICU is full of abnormal numbers. The ICU is full of patients who are very sick and need aggressive interventions. It is very easy to make those abnormal numbers go away. That does not mean that I have done the patient a favor or treated them appropriately. I can "do everything" to a patient who comes to my ICU. That does not mean I have fulfilled that patient's goals of care. We need to always treat the patient, and sometimes that may mean doing nothing at all.

CHAPTER 5
ICU RULE NUMBER NINE

Everything that could go wrong with this patient went wrong during this hospital stay. She had cancer, and she underwent several rounds of chemotherapy. This round was supposed to be the easiest of all the cycles. For some reason, however, this round was the absolute worst. The chemo levels refused to go down, unlike her previous rounds. The complications of the chemotherapy — mouth sores, nausea, and diarrhea — were SO MUCH worse this time around. She even threw up blood on several occasions. And soon after the chemo finished, the fevers started…and they never stopped.

They were relentless. No matter how much medication was prescribed, the fevers never went below 100 degrees. And with the fevers came the body aches, the fast breathing, and the fast heart rate. She really got sick, but she was always stable. Her oxygen levels would sometimes go down quite significantly, but she was still stable. Her blood pressure still stayed normal. And there was the pain. She was in so much pain. She knew the name of the pain medicine, Dilaudid, by name. She asked for it every two hours like clockwork.

She was like this for almost a week, and then suddenly, early in the morning on a Saturday, something changed. She was much less responsive. Her breathing became much more labored, and she seemed to have more phlegm and junk in her lungs than before. It was not long before her blood pressure — heretofore the best thing about her vital signs — began to drop like a rock.

Despite getting plenty of IV fluids, the blood pressure continued to decrease. So, a blood pressure medication called dopamine was started. Her renal function continued to deteriorate, despite getting multiple blood products to try and further support the blood pressure. Her breathing became even worse, and she was placed on noninvasive mechanical ventilation. By that night, she had to be placed on a ventilator, and it was clear that she went into acute renal failure and would require dialysis.

The shock would continue to get worse, and multiple other blood pressure medications – called vasopressors – were added, in vain, to keep the blood pressure elevated. The patient was gasping for air, even though she was on the ventilator. Her feet were mottled and blue, meaning that the circulation was shutting down. Her fingers were blue. She was still burning up from fever. There was very little urine in the urine collection bag. I knew it was not good. It was clear that the patient was going to die.

The family, having been told that their loved one would likely die, elected to continue treatment at the same level, but not escalate care further. She would not be resuscitated in case of cardiac arrest. Soon after this, the heart rate started to slowly go down: 200, 190, 180, 170, 160, 150, 140. I wondered how long it would be, but then suddenly, the heart rate went from 140 to zero, and the patient passed away.

That patient was my 12-year-old daughter. She died on June 7, 2009, a day forever burned into my memory. She was killed by gram-negative septic shock causing multiorgan failure.

This story brings me to **ICU Rule Number Nine**:

BE CAREFUL WITH THE WORDS, "LOOK I UNDERSTAND."

Every day, in every ICU across the world, similar stories of tragedy and grief occur. Every day, in every ICU across the world, parents lose their children; children lose their parents; and so many other relationships are shattered by critical illness. These tragedies increased many fold during the COVID-19 pandemic. As clinicians caring for these patients – and watching their loved ones grieve – we feel a need to try and help those left behind, we feel a need to try and comfort those having to deal with the loss of a loved one in the ICU.

But, if we say, "*Look, I understand,*" we need to ask ourselves: do we *really* understand? Do we *really* understand what they are experiencing? At the about the same time as my daughter died, another colleague lost her daughter – in her 30s and the prime of life – to brain cancer. She was as devastated as I was. She told me once, remarking about the priest speaking during a memorial service, "*What does he understand about what I'm going through?*" It is a natural question.

It is a difficult balance to maintain. When we give bad news to a patient's family member – like the doctors gave my wife and me about our daughter – the medical logic may be perfect. For example, I had a patient who suffered a catastrophic brain injury, and it was unlikely that she would ever wake up again. To me, as an ICU doctor, it is completely logical and rational.

To a loved one, however, those words are absolutely devastating. Telling a daughter that her mother will never wake up is just as catastrophic as the initial brain injury. Telling a mother and father that their son will need to live on a ventilator for weeks, if not months, or that their son will not survive, is equally catastrophic. As the clinician giving this news, it is sometimes hard to see how catastrophic those words truly are.

On the one hand, I need to be objective and rational, not taken in by the emotion of the moment, so I can explain the medicine as cogently and completely as I can. It is important that I give my patients' families accurate facts and data, so we can all make the most informed medical decision possible. On the other hand, when I am totally enveloped in the medicine and its logic, it can be hard to see why what I am saying is causing so much distress on the part of the family. "*What is so hard to understand or accept?*" I may ask myself. "*The medical logic is absolutely concrete and linear.*"

But, when giving bad news to family, I am no longer in the realm of "medical logic." I am in the realm of emotion, devastation and catastrophe. Families cling to every single word I say, and sometimes they are trying to hold on to any semblance of hope in my words. It can be hard to fully understand this, and this is where we doctors are liable to come off as callous and uncaring.

Which is why I, when giving bad news to a family member or loved one, always share the story of my daughter. I am not looking for any sort of sympathy, even though I am always given words of comfort. Rather, I am letting them know that I *truly do understand* what they are going through. I *truly have been* in a similar situation. And, almost always, it has helped me connect with the family and help them process the horrific experience of having a loved one be critically ill and die.

I am *not* saying do not show any sympathy or empathy. I *am* saying be careful with uttering the words, "Look, I understand" – unless you truly do understand. When they were putting dirt over my daughter's pink casket, I was overwhelmed by the situation and openly sobbed at her gravesite. Someone came up from behind me and said, "Be patient." It was the "right words" to say in that situation, and it backfired. I wanted to turn around and scream to him, "Let me grieve, for God's sake!!!" I didn't, but I so wanted to.

Sometimes, words of empathy – even if genuine – may not be helpful, and so, if you have also suffered from a similar tragedy, I would encourage you to share it with patients' families, if you are comfortable doing so. First, similar to my experience, you can develop a connection with the patient's family on a much deeper level. You can help them deal with the tragedy of the death of their loved one. Second, it may help you deal with your own grief and sadness. It has surely helped me: it has made me see that the death of my daughter – as unimaginably horrific as it has been – continues to bring goodness into the world. Her death continues to bring others life and love, and that is very comforting for me.

In the ICU, we are truly fighting – literally and figuratively – a bloody battle with critical illness. We fight like hell until either we win, or the fight cannot be won despite our every effort. Let us always be cognizant of the fact that our patients' families are watching that fight with horror, fear and trepidation. When it is time to give bad news, let us remember how devastating our "medically logical" words can be to them and deliver those words with the utmost care and compassion. And just be cognizant of the fact that the words, "Look, I understand," may not be as helpful as they were intended to be.

CHAPTER 6
ICU RULE NUMBER TEN

"*Are you sure you don't want to replace the potassium?*

"*Yes, I'm sure.*"

"*Are you sure?*"

"*Yes, I'm sure.*"

"*Okaaayyy...you're the doctor.*"

I cannot, in polite company and on the pages of this book, relay what the next two words I would really want to say after the above exchange with an ICU nurse are.

Of course, I jest. Yet, I cannot tell you how many times an ICU nurse would say those words to me, also in gest. When I first rotated in the ICU as an intern, I had already decided that Critical Care Medicine was what I wanted to be when I "grew up." Yet, little did I know how much growing up I really needed when I first arrived there.

I came down to the ICU thinking I was God's gift to Critical Care. "*Hey ICU!*" I thought to myself, "*Dr. Hassaballa has arrived!*" I came down the ICU roaring like a lion. It only took four weeks for me to leave the ICU rotation meowing like a little kitten. And who was it that transformed me from a lion to a kitten? The ICU nurses.

I still remember the time I finished placing a central line on a patient. I walked out the ICU room saying, "OK guys, thanks so much!"

"Umm…excuse me!" said the ICU nurse in the room.

I stopped dead in my tracks, confused.

"What?" I replied.

"Where are you going?"

Baffled, I replied, "Uh…to the nurses' station to write the procedure note." I truly did not understand what the problem was.

"The sharps? Are you going to put them away?" said the nurse back to me, incredulous, at my confusion.

"The sharps" are the needles and sutures we leave behind after placing the central line into the major vein in the neck. I walked out of the room thinking the nurses would put them away for me. I chuckle at this now thinking about at how stupid I was.

"Oh…uh…sure, I will do it," I say, sheepishly coming back to the room and putting away the "sharps" into the designated container in the room.

Obviously, that was the absolute right thing to do. Obviously, I can't leave my sharp needles and sutures for the nurses to clean up and then potentially get hurt and exposed to a patient's blood and body fluids. Obviously, making sure the nurses are safe when they take care of our patients is paramount. As a dumb intern, however, that was clearly not obvious enough for me, and the ICU nurses made sure I learned the lesson.

ICU nurses are among the most – if not the most – highly skilled bedside clinicians in the hospital. They know their stuff, and they are not afraid to share their opinions with the doctors when they do not agree, especially the experienced ICU nurses. More often than not, their "gut feelings" are right on the money, and it is not a good idea to ignore their instincts.

And this is why ICU nurses are the subject of my **ICU Rule Number Ten**:

NEVER CROSS AN ICU NURSE

Just never do it.

If you treat the ICU nurses poorly; if you think – like I did – that you are God's gift to Critical Care; if you disrespect the ICU nurses because *you* are a Doctor, and *they* are just a nurse; if you do that, first of all it is rude and highly inappropriate. As importantly, if you treat them badly, they are apt to make your life very difficult in the ICU.

Remember all those abnormal numbers in the ICU, many of which are clinically insignificant? Treat the ICU nurses poorly, and you will get called for every single one of those abnormal numbers because, "you're the Doctor," and you need to know about them.

Treat the ICU nurses poorly, and they will continue to bother you with things they know are not important, all the while apologizing and saying – with a straight face – "I'm sorry to bother you, Doctor." Treating the ICU nurses poorly creates a terrible tension that can destroy the culture of the ICU.

But more than just self-preservation in the ICU, treating the ICU nurses poorly can place patient care at risk. Critical Care is a team sport, and every member of the team – the ICU nurse chief among them – contributes to the care of the patient. If your attitude and demeanor is such that the members of the care team – the ICU nurses chief among them – avoid approaching you because you are a total jerk, you are only hurting the patient. This is unacceptable.

The ICU nurses are your most important patient care ally; the ICU nurses are at the patient's bedside the entire day, much more than we are, even if we only practice in the ICU. They have much more insight into how the patients are doing. I take what they tell me very seriously, and when they say to me, "*Hassaballa, get into the room and look at this patient*," I listen immediately, because they would not say this if they did not feel the patient warranted my attention.

When patients are delirious, sometimes they will physically attack the ICU nurses, injuring them in the process. This is totally unacceptable to me. While, yes, patient safety is #1 in the hospital, staff safety is – to me – #1b.

I learned to respect and appreciate the ICU nurses during my first rotation in the ICU, and even though they taught me humility the hard way, I am forever grateful, because it made me an exponentially better ICU physician. I am forever grateful because, I would not be as successful in the ICU without the ICU nurses. Whenever I start working in an ICU, I make sure I treat the ICU nurses extra special, frequently getting them coffee or bagels or doughnuts, or lunch. They deserve to be treated extra special, because they are the heart of the ICU and the life-saving care we provide to our patients there.

And…in the wake of the horrors of the COVID-19 pandemic, I am forever in awe of what I witnessed them do at the bedside for those patients afflicted with that terrible illness. Nowadays, COVID may not be that big of a deal. But, in the Spring of 2020, it was an absolute nightmare. So many ICUs around the country – including my own – were inundated with patient after patient with this mysterious viral illness for which we had no treatment and which was killing people day in and day out.

All of us were filled with fear of this mysterious illness; fear that the illness will afflict us and take our lives – or even worse – the lives of our families. So many of us, myself included, would refuse to hug our children when we came home after our shift until we took off our scrubs (frequently in the garage) and showered thoroughly. So many of us, myself included, would sleep away from our families for fear of spreading this illness unbeknownst to them. So many of us were terrified of taking care of COVID patients, but take care of them we did, because it was our duty as clinicians in the ICU.

And the ICU nurses were at the center of that care. They had that fear just like everyone else, but they put that fear aside and spent their entire shift at the bedside of these horribly sick patients. They would not even leave to eat or use the restroom because they were afraid of what would happen if they were not there. The PPE, or personal protective equipment, would create physical deformities on their faces because they would have to wear them for hours upon hours without a break.

And when the patients would die – and die by the millions they did – the ICU nurses would refuse to have them die alone, especially in the beginning of the pandemic when we restricted visitation from family members. I will never forget – and will forever be in total admiration of them for this – watching them hold the hands of the patients dying from COVID, with the family screaming in agony on an iPad. If there was ever a hero in the ICU during the COVID pandemic, it was the ICU nurse, hands down.

To all the ICU nurses reading this, all I can say is: Thank You. Thank you for your dedication. Thank you for your passion for our patients. Thank you for your heart, your grit, and your tenacity. Thank you for all you did for our patients during the dark times of the COVID pandemic. Thank you for your relentless pursuit of doing right by our patients. Thank you for teaching me humility as an intern and making me a much, much better physician. If I filled this entire book with the words "Thank You," it would still not fully encapsulate how grateful I am for you. Thank you, thank you, thank you.

CHAPTER 7
ICU RULE NUMBER ELEVEN

It was my turn to work the Thanksgiving holiday. Fortunately, the shift went by smoothly. I had seen all of my patients, taken care of everything they needed, and was hanging out in the ICU waiting for my shift to end without incident. My family was gathering at my Aunt's house for Thanksgiving dinner, and I was looking forward to a wonderful meal and a wonderful evening with my extended family. Moreover, the Bears were playing the Packers that day, and I could not wait to watch the game with all of my cousins. And, if the Bears won (a rare occurrence, I admit,) I would get to rub it into my wife, who is a diehard Packer fan. So, quitting time could not come soon enough.

Alas, it would not come to be. Fifteen minutes before my shift ended, a patient unfortunately suffered cardiac arrest. I urgently went to the bedside, ran the code, and then transferred the patient to the ICU. I then proceeded to spend almost 2 hours with the patient: performing procedures and stabilizing the clinical situation. All the while, my family – which was waiting for me literally in the car to come home so we could go to my aunt's house – was making multiple phone calls to my cell phone wondering where I was. Finally, my wife called the ICU and asked if I was there, and they answered in the affirmative. I was able to eventually leave, but I missed all of the good food when we finally arrived at my aunt's house for dinner.

This sort of situation has happened to me more times than I

would like to recount throughout my career in the ICU. I could be twiddling my thumbs the entire day, and then, all of a sudden, a patient somewhere deteriorates, and I spend hour upon hour at that patient's bedside. Not infrequently, I have to stay after my shift ends. It is a fact of life, not only in critical care, but in medicine in general. And it highlights my **ICU Rule Number Eleven**:

THE ONLY PREDICTABLE THING ABOUT THE ICU IS THAT IT IS UNPREDICTABLE.

Critical illness can creep up on you without any notice. So often, the patient in the ICU will be sick, but stable throughout the day, and then all of a sudden – without warning – that patient will suffer a life-threatening arrhythmia, or will develop sudden shock, or will have a complication related to the underlying illness, or emergently need to go on a ventilator. And then, we have to quickly act and intervene to prevent the patient from dying.

During my training, I was working at a long-term care facility and had two patients suffer cardiac arrest…at the exact same time. And, I was literally running between both rooms running both codes at once. During the depths of the COVID pandemic, I had an entire ICU filled with super sick patients suffering multiple unpredictable complications all at once. It was not uncommon for me to also run between two or three rooms, shouting out orders to treat this complication, or that. It was really a terrible time.

Many patients in the ICU are a ticking time bomb, and they can explode at any moment without any warning. That is why they are in the ICU in the first place, and the ICU is the only place equipped to handle sudden and unpredictable deterioration. And, just like timing the stock market, it is folly to try to predict when these complications will happen.

We can start the day in the ICU with just a few patients, and then before we know it, we will have seen seven new patients within a span of a few hours. That is what happened during COVID. Despite having an ICU completely filled with COVID patients on ventilators, any number of patients on the floors outside of the ICU were on the brink of life-threatening collapse. And you could never predict who was the next one to go down and need our attention.

Yes, this predictable unpredictability has caused me to miss countless dinners, has caused me to be late to countless gatherings, and has ruined countless evening plans with my family. Not uncommonly, as I am literally walking out of the hospital, a patient will suffer cardiac arrest, and I have to turn around and come back to the hospital. I have even left the hospital, and then had to turn around my car and go back. And, yes, none of this is predictable.

No doubt, it can be very stressful. Of course, it would be nice to be absolutely certain that, at the end of my shift, I'm going to be able to go home on time. And most of the times, in many if not most ICUs around the country, there is a clinician on duty 24 hours a day, and so when your partner comes in, you can safely leave. But, sometimes, there is only one person covering the ICU at one time. Or, despite the presence of your partner, you still have to stay and take care of things left over from the shift.

No doubt, this predictable unpredictability can get old. No doubt, I have become frustrated so many times when, just as I am looking forward to taking a break, another patient emergency occurs, and I have to get up and run all over again. Heck, it was like that almost nonstop during the dark times of COVID.

But if we recognize that this is part of the deal, if we recognize that critical illness is inherently unpredictable, then we can be prepared. Perhaps one of the things that can overwhelm people who are not used to working in the ICU is this predictable unpredictability. So many people are shocked that a patient can seem stable the entire day, and then all of a sudden actively try to die in a matter of minutes, forcing you to drop everything and focus your attention solely on that person. That is indeed what makes the ICU difficult.

But it is also what makes the ICU exhilarating. When that inevitable predictable unpredictability strikes, you are able to act quickly on your feet and intervene to save a patient's life. And when your intervention stabilizes the patient and prevents them from dying, the feeling this gives is truly indescribable. It's why I became a doctor in the first place: to help people get better and survive their illness.

When we recognize that this can happen at any moment, without warning, then it should not stress us out. And when that predictable, unpredictability strikes, the most important thing is not to panic. This is why "Don't Panic" is my top rule of the ICU (and rules number two through five, as well).

And so, knowing that the only predictable thing in the ICU is that it is unpredictable, we need to take the lulls when they come. Yes, it can get crazy busy for hours on end. But it can also be crazy slow for hours on end as well. It can be crazy slow for days on end, just like it can be crazy busy for days on end. Whenever those slow times come, I will take full advantage of them.

That is when I write. That is when I do research. That is when I perform administrative tasks. That is when I walk around the ICU and listen to music. The lulls are gifts from God to allow me to rest, recuperate, and recharge for the next inevitable patient deterioration.

Indeed, persistently slow time is in the ICU may give my business colleagues palpitations. And, indeed, as Director of the ICU, a long stretch of slow days makes me nervous as well. But this is the time for me not to panic because, I know that eventually, it will get busy all of a sudden. I know that the predictable unpredictability of the ICU will always prevail. And so, I live every second of the slow times.

Therefore, I recommend you do the same. As long as it is safe from a patient care perspective, try to do something you enjoy: writing, drawing, listening to music, having coffee with colleagues…anything to relax the mind.

No doubt, this is easier for me to do as the ICU physician rather than an ICU nurse with a very sick patient. Yet, this is where I see the ICU nurses chip in to help each other take that well-deserved break so they can decompress and recharge. This is also why I am full of admiration for them. This is so important, and I recommend every ICU in the country have some sort of process to allow bedside clinicians a break throughout the shift.

Clinician burnout has reached alarming levels, and it has been accelerated by the COVID-19 pandemic. Physicians commit suicide at a rate much higher than the general population. This is truly a crisis.

The underlying causes are multifactorial, and there is no doubt that the stresses of our jobs today have a big influence on causing this burnout. But also, the ever-increasing burden of paperwork and administrative tasks that get in the way of bedside patient care are also a major factor. It needs to be addressed on a systemic level because, if there are no more clinicians caring for our patients because they have burned out and left the field - which is happening currently in droves - or they are caring for patients while being burned out, then it is truly a catastrophe.

I also think that part of what may fuel burn out is a mismatch in expectations. Expecting to work in an ICU, with critically ill patients, and have nothing happen all of a sudden is unrealistic. This is not how critically-ill patients behave. And, after the COVID-19 pandemic, the patients being admitted to the ICU are only going to be sicker and so the predictable unpredictability is only going to be more predictable.

Therefore, we need to reset our expectations. We need to recognize that, at any moment, we are going to become crazy busy for hours on end. That is part of the deal. Therefore, when the lulls come, when the slow times arrive, take absolutely full advantage. Don't ever sweat the slow times because, they are not going to last forever.

EPILOGUE

I was called to evaluate a patient sick with COVID-19 on the medical floor. She was a breast cancer patient, getting chemotherapy. When I first saw her, she was literally on the floor, gasping for air. We helped her back to her bed, and we decided she needed to be transferred emergently to the ICU. She continued to deteriorate, and she ended up needing a ventilator. For patients with COVID-19, especially in the very beginning of the pandemic, going on a ventilator was frequently a death sentence.

There was another patient for whom I was caring in May 2020. He was 43-year-old, also sick with COVID-19. His oxygen levels were dangerously low, and he needed a lot of support with pressure and oxygen to make sure his levels remained normal. The team and I was watching him very closely, because any sign of distress would mean he would need to go on a ventilator. So far, he was holding his own. Again, going on a ventilator frequently meant death, and I did not take this decision lightly.

By the next day, however, things became a little worse. While he was still talking to me and able to interact with us – albeit in a tight-fitting mask – there were subtle signs of distress, and I did not want him to struggle more, which can cause lung damage in and of itself. And so, I decided to intubate and place him on a ventilator. I got all dressed up in my PPE, said a prayer, and then entered his room.

The set up for the intubation was routine, and once everything was ready, I said another prayer and proceeded with intubation. The procedure went very smoothly. That was not the problem. It was afterwards that something went wrong.

I was absolutely sure the tube went into the lungs. Despite this, his lungs were not moving properly on the machine. His oxygen levels were still low. We then took him off the ventilator and breathed for him manually. His oxygen levels finally came up, and I was relieved. Then, suddenly, his heart rate slowed down and then stopped altogether.

We called a "CODE BLUE." I immediately got on his chest myself and did CPR. We gave multiple drugs to jump-start his heart. It worked, thank God, and his heart came back, and he even opened his eyes. I was so relieved.

There were a number of procedures I was planning to perform to help him get treatment, and as I was setting up for them, his oxygen decreased again. I started working with the ventilator, trying to do what I could to help bring them up. Then, his heart stopped again. We called another "CODE BLUE."

We did CPR, we gave multiple drugs, we worked and worked and worked and worked on him. We did everything possible to try to bring him back. We were not successful. He died despite all that we did.

As the CODE BLUE was proceeding, I was getting the sinking feeling that he was not going to survive. I was praying for him silently. You could see the anguish on my face. I was trying to keep it together, because there were a lot of other very sick patients in the ICU that needed my care.

My heart sank again knowing I had to call his wife and tell her the horrific news. She was devastated.

"I don't understand," she said. "They told me he was doing OK yesterday."

"He *was* doing OK yesterday," I replied. "Sometimes, these things happen and we don't understand why." I couldn't say sorry enough times.

Right at that moment, I got the news that the hospital was about to discharge a patient who had suffered cardiac arrest and survived despite all the odds working against her. I helped take care of her, and I needed that moment of positivity after such a terrible incident. As I was walking out of the ICU, I saw one of the nurses who was helping us in the code.

"Thank you for all your help," I said, barely able to say the words, tears welling up in my eyes.

"Are you OK?" she asked.

"Yeah, I'm OK," I replied.

But, I was not OK. Then, all of the sudden, as the ICU doors opened and I walked out to a large crowd of people waiting for the survivor to leave, I lost it and openly and loudly sobbed. I couldn't stand, overcome with the emotion and anguish and distress of what had just happened.

Multiple people came over to comfort me, and I was able to stop crying. I got to see our patient – blowing kisses to the dozens of staff, including me, clapping and cheering for her – leave the hospital alive and well. I got multiple texts of support from friends and colleagues. The following morning, on my computer in the ICU, someone had put a sign saying: "*Hang in there my friend…we're all in this together!!! We got this.*" The support I received was truly wonderful, and it helped ease the pain of that day. I still have this sign behind the computer more than two years later.

This patient was not the first patient I had lost in the ICU. He was not the first patient I had lost to COVID-19. This time, however, it was different. His loss hit me particularly hard, and I couldn't stop the emotions from flowing out of me.

I will not lie: I thought about leaving the bedside during the depths of the COVID-19 pandemic. Despite how much I loved working in the ICU; despite all the fun I have working in the ICU, I seriously considered leaving the bedside. I had ample opportunity to work clinical jobs remotely, and I would not have to worry about risking my life taking care of sick people during this – or any inevitable future – pandemic.

The pull to that bedside, however, was too strong. I could not bring myself to do it. As I mentioned in the very beginning, there is nothing else I ever wanted to be except a physician. It was the only thing of which I had ever dreamed. Any other career would have been a compromise. So, leaving the bedside for good was just too much for me to bear.

Sure, as I get older, I am more tired. No doubt, the night shifts are getting old. No doubt, the sleep deprivation that comes with night shifts is also getting old. There will be one day that I will finally make the decision and leave the bedside for good.

May of 2020 was not that day. Indeed, that day has not yet arrived in 2023, and I do not think it will arrive for the foreseeable future. The pull to the bedside is just too strong.

And so, dear reader, I urge you to step back and take it all in. In 2010 – on October 10, to be exact (10/10/10) – I ran the Chicago Marathon in honor of my daughter who passed away the year before after losing her battle with cancer. I was super nervous – I had previously gotten tired driving 26.2 miles, let alone running them – and I did not know how the race would go, whether I would even finish. My cousin, who was running with me, told me, "Take it all in."

We should do the same with Medicine. Take it all in. It is not cliché to say that Medicine is a calling, not just a field. It is a call to care for people at their most vulnerable – when they are afflicted with illness. It is a calling to put the well-being of others ahead of yourself. It is a calling to help relieve the suffering of complete strangers, who place their trust in us to help them in their time of need.

And the path to answer that calling is fraught with difficulty. One can argue it is made too difficult, actually, but difficult it is nonetheless. And so for those of us who were gifted to be able to answer that calling, like me, we should step back and take in that blessed reality.

You are a nurse; you are a respiratory therapist, physical therapist, occupational therapist; you are a nutritionist; and, you are a doctor. You care for the ill; you help relieve their suffering; you help people overcome their illness and feel better. This is a very special thing, and we should not only take it all in, but we should never take it for granted.

Sure, there are problems – major problems – with our healthcare system. Yes, the pandemic has exacerbated healthcare inequities and exposed them for all to see. Yes, clinicians are faced with tremendous challenges and stresses navigating healthcare today. And in the aftermath of the COVID-19 scourge, droves of healers have left our field for other pursuits, adding to the challenges we have to face.

Despite all of this, I am still so very grateful I am a physician.

Despite all of the annoyances with which I must deal as a physician – especially a physician in the ICU – I am still so very grateful that I called Rush Medical College that May morning in 1995 and asked about my status on the waiting list. I am still so very grateful that I get to help people conquer life-threatening critical illness, and if I can't conquer their illness, then help minimize their suffering and provide them a "good death," a death with dignity and comfort. I am so very grateful to be given this opportunity and each and every day.

And so, dear reader, take it all in. As we ran the Chicago Marathon, it was very difficult. The weather was hot. As I crossed the 22 mile mark, I could barely walk, let alone run. My entire body was in pain. But never, not even once, did I think about stopping the race and calling it quits. If I had to finish crawling across the finish line, then so be it. I had to do this for my daughter, who I knew was sitting on top of the "Finish" sign, smiling, and waiting for me to finish the race in her honor. I took in the race, even its most difficult moments, and when I was done, it was one of the happiest moments of my entire life. The medal they put around my neck is the most precious inanimate object I own.

When we are done with the marathon of our career in healthcare, it is my hope that we will be just as happy. When we are done with the marathon of our career in healthcare, while we may have carried many a scar along the way, it is my hope that we will have helped so many people while getting those scars. When we are done with the marathon of our career in healthcare, we may not have a medal to take home with us, but we will have the knowledge that we have made the world a better place by answering the calling to heal the sick.

One day, I will finally leave the bedside. But, until that day comes, I will take in and enjoy every moment on the journey. I hope and pray, dear colleague, that you do the very same.

APPENDIX

HONORING THE ORGAN DONOR

This is the prayer I wrote honoring those patients who give the gift of life to others by donating one or more organs. Whenever I get the chance, I read it in the hospital as the patient is wheeled out of the ICU for the last time.

Lord our God, God of Hope, God of Healing, God of Life:

You gave me this body, and You gave me my soul
That I may walk and breathe and live
Now You have called me back to become whole
And so my body, as a gift, I now give

I tried to live a life that was best
To spread Your Peace and do none harm
And now that I am to be laid to rest
Please, O Lord, embrace me in your Arms

I pray, O Lord, my heart does not fail
So that Your child can live and love
I pray, O Lord, my lungs always sail
So that Your child can breathe from above

I pray, O Lord, my liver runs along
To keep Your child sane and whole
I pray, O Lord, my kidneys sing their song
And let Your child laugh and console

And if, O Lord, I cannot give all You Gave
I pray that You bless whatever was saved

Now please, O Lord, comfort my beloved
Lord, bring them ease from their pain
Please, O Lord, look after my beloved
And shower Your Care like the rain

Also, O Lord, bless the ones who received
The gift I passed from You to they
Give them the grace of stress relieved
And to them Your Peace do I convey

In Your Most Holy Name do I pray this. Amen.

ABOUT THE AUTHOR

Hesham Hassaballa, MD, FCCP, FAASM is a New York Times-featured practicing Pulmonary and Critical Care Medicine physician. He is board certified in Internal Medicine, Pulmonary Medicine, Critical Care, and Sleep Medicine. Dr. Hassaballa is a Regional Medical Director, leading and overseeing clinical operations in multiple ICUs in the across the country.

Dr. Hassaballa is an Assistant Professor of Medicine and Course Director for Rush University Medical Center, Assistant Professor of Medicine for the University of Tennessee Health Sciences Center College of Medicine, and Adjunct Assistant Professors of Medicine for Drexel University College of Medicine. He serves as a peer reviewer for the Society of Critical Care Medicine. He has presented research a number of times at national meetings, and he has published numerous articles in peer-reviewed medical journals.

Dr. Hassaballa has won a number of awards, most recently a Core Value Award for Teamwork, a Medical Staff Leadership Award along with a Promise and Humanitarian Award at the hospital in which he currently practices.

In addition to his clinical and administrative roles, Dr. Hassaballa serves as Treasurer of the Bayan Hassaballa Foundation, set up by he and his wife to honor the memory of their daughter, Bayan, who lost her battle with cancer in 2009 (www.ourangelbayan.org).

Dr. Hassaballa's writing can be found at www.drhassaballa.com and www.healthcaremusings.com.

Made in the USA
Monee, IL
08 November 2026

67378662R00035